Clinical Research and Case Report On Cardiovascular Disease by Pharmacists in Japan

Heart Failure and Disseminated Intravascular Coagulation

Yuki Asai

ELIVA PRESS

ELIVA PRESS

Yuki Asai

Pharmacists need to conduct clinical research and case reports as drug experts. This time, we indicated a case report in which a pharmacist proposed a combination therapy of midodrine and droxidopa to a doctor for refractory hypotension in a patient with chronic heart failure. In addition, we showed the results of a retrospective study evaluating the efficacy of recombinant human soluble thrombomodulin, a therapeutic agent for disseminated intravascular coagulation.

Published by Eliva Press SRL
Address: MD-2060, bd.Cuza-Voda, 1/4, of. 21 Chişinău, Republica
Moldova
Email: info@elivapress.com
Website: www.elivapress.com

ISBN: 978-1-63648-151-7

Author

Yuki Asai Ph. D (Pharmacy)

Preface

Pharmacists should actively conduct clinical researches and case reports as a drug expert. This time, we report a case report and a retrospective study conducted mainly by pharmacists.

Contents

Chapter 1
Factors influencing the effectiveness of recombinant human soluble thrombomodulin on disseminated intravascular coagulation: a retrospective study

Chapter 2
Combination therapy of midodrine and droxidopa for refractory hypotension in heart failure with preserved ejection fraction per a pharmacist's proposal: a case report

Chapter 1

Factors influencing the effectiveness of recombinant human soluble thrombomodulin on disseminated intravascular coagulation: a retrospective study

Authors

Yuki Asai, Takanori Yamamoto, Daisuke Kito, Kazuya Ichikawa, Yasuharu Abe

Abstract

Background: Although recombinant human soluble thrombomodulin (rTM) has been widely used to treat disseminated intravascular coagulation (DIC) in Japan, there is no consensus regarding rTM efficacy. Therefore, if the factors influencing rTM efficacy is revealed, it may be possible to demonstrate the effectiveness of rTM by limiting the patients who use rTM. This study investigated the factors of rTM treatment which influence DIC status.

Methods: This retrospective case-control study enrolled hospitalized adult patients treated with rTM from October 2010 to May 2020. Among these patients, 227 who were diagnosed with DIC according to the Japanese

Association for Acute Medicine DIC scoring system were assessed. The primary endpoint was the 28-day mortality after rTM treatment. For Cox-proportional hazards model, explanatory factors determined using univariate analysis with $p < 0.1$ were used. In addition, some factors considered to affect DIC-related mortality such as age $\geq$ 75 years, rTM dose $\geq$ 380 U/kg, antithrombin III treatment, and diseases with a poor prognosis (sepsis, solid tumors, and trauma) were added as covariates.

Results: Univariate analyses suggested that male sex ($p = 0.029$), treatment in intensive care unit ($p = 0.061$), and prothrombin time-international normalized ratio (PT-INR) ($p < 0.001$) were the factors influencing DIC-related 28-day mortality after rTM treatment. According to Cox-proportional hazard analysis, the adjusted odds ratio for DIC-related 28-day mortality in patients with PT-INR $\geq$ 1.67 was 2.23 (95% confidence interval: 1.451–3.433, $p < 0.001$), age $\geq$ 75 years was 1.57 (95% confidence interval: 1.009–2.439, $p = 0.046$), and male sex was 1.66 (95% confidence interval: 1.065–2.573, $p = 0.025$), respectively. As life-threatening bleeding events were not observed, prolonged PT-INR might directly or indirectly affect DIC-related mortality caused by rTM treatment.

5

Conclusion: rTM treatment for DIC was less effective in male patients with PT-

INR ≥ 1.67 and age ≥ 75 years.

Background

Disseminated intravascular coagulation (DIC) is among the most common emergency conditions and is characterized by organ damage because of microvascular obstruction by excessive thrombin production [1]. Simultaneous administration of platelets and coagulation factors leads to systemic hemorrhage. Because DIC is associated with high mortality, both early diagnosis and appropriate therapy are essential to improve patient outcomes [2].

Thrombomodulin (TM) is a protein that binds with high affinity to thrombin and protein C receptor, thus performing an important role in regulating coagulation [3]. Activated protein C produced following controlled degradation of the thrombin-TM complex inhibits thrombin generation by degrading and inactivating the coagulation factors VIIIa and V [4]. Recombinant human soluble thrombomodulin (rTM), a novel anticoagulant, has been widely used to improve DIC status in Japan [5-7]. Recently, Saito *et al.* [5] revealed no significant differences in DIC resolution rates following rTM treatment and heparin treatment; they also demonstrated that bleeding events following rTM treatment were lower than following heparin treatment. Although rTM treatment is highly effective and safe according to many studies [5-7], a randomized, double-blind, multinational, multicenter phase 3 study (SCARLET Randomized Clinical Trial) has reported no significant differences in 28-day mortality rate following rTM therapy and that following placebo therapy [8]. Consequently, there is no consensus on the effectiveness of rTM because some factors could affect the research results. Therefore, revealing the factors influencing rTM efficacy may help in demonstrating the effectiveness of rTM by limiting the patients receiving rTM.

The aim of the present study was to determine the factors influencing DIC-related mortality in patients after rTM treatment.

Methods

Subjects

This single-center, retrospective case-control study was performed at the National Hospital Organization Mie Chuo Medical Center (Mie, Japan), using electronic medical records. Herein, DIC was evaluated using the diagnostic criteria specified by the Japanese Association for Acute Medicine (JAAM) DIC scoring system (Table 1) [9]. DIC was diagnosed when the JAAM DIC score exceeded 4 points. We selected 251 adult, hospitalized patients treated with rTM from October 2010 to May 2020. Among these patients, 227 patients diagnosed with DIC were enrolled.

Baseline characteristics

The primary outcome was 28-day mortality after rTM treatment. We classified patients into survival and death groups based on whether they survived for 28 days. Baseline clinical characteristics and laboratory data that were examined in parallel to rTM treatment (Table 2).

Statistical analysis

As previous studies reported that the 28-day mortality after rTM treatment was lesser than 40 [8,11], we expected a minimum 28-day mortality rate of 40%

after rTM treatment. Considering 90% power for this study and a significance level of 0.05, sample size was calculated as 182 per group. Continuous variables were compared between the survival and death groups using Student's t-test or Mann–Whitney U test. Fisher's exact test was conducted to compare categorical variables between the groups. The overall survival rate was calculated using Kaplan–Meier estimator and compared using the log-rank test. The missing value of PT-INR in the survival (n = 2) and death groups (n = 2) were replaced by the median values of each group, respectively. Multivariate analysis was conducted using the Cox-proportional hazards model. For Cox-proportional hazards model, explanatory factors determined using univariate analysis with $p < 0.1$ were used. Furthermore, some factors considered to affect DIC-related mortality including age ≥ 75 years [12], rTM dose ≥ 380 U/kg [13], ATIII treatment [11], and diseases with a poor prognosis (sepsis, solid tumors, and trauma) [1] were added as covariates. Moreover, the cutoff value for the extracted continuous variables calculated from receiver operating characteristic (ROC) analysis was used (Fig. 1). Statistical analyses were performed using EZR software (Saitama Medical Center, Jichi Medical University, Saitama, Japan) [14] with significance established at $p < 0.05$.

Results

The proportion of patients with the subtype of diseases that caused DIC, such as sepsis, solid tumors, and trauma, was shown in Table 2, but the proportion was not statistically different between the survival and death groups. The 28-day mortality rate after rTM treatment was 45.4% (124/227 patients). Univariate analysis revealed that male sex (p = 0.029), treatment in ICU (p = 0.061), and PT-INR (p < 0.001) are possible factors influencing DIC-related 28-day mortality after rTM treatment (Table 2). The PT-INR cutoff value was 1.45 which corresponds to the results of the ROC analysis (sensitivity: 73%, specificity: 53%, area under the curve: 0.65) (Fig. 1). Figure 2 displays Kaplan–Meier curves for 28-day mortality after rTM treatment in patients with PT-INR < 1.67 and PT-INR ≥ 1.67. The adjusted odds ratio for 28-day mortality in patients with PT-INR ≥ 1.67 was 2.23 (95% confidence interval: 1.451–3.433, p < 0.001), age ≥ 75 years was 1.57 (95% confidence interval: 1.009–2.439, p = 0.046), and male sex was 1.66 (95% confidence interval: 1.065–2.573, p = 0.025). Life-threatening bleeding events were not observed in the mortality group.

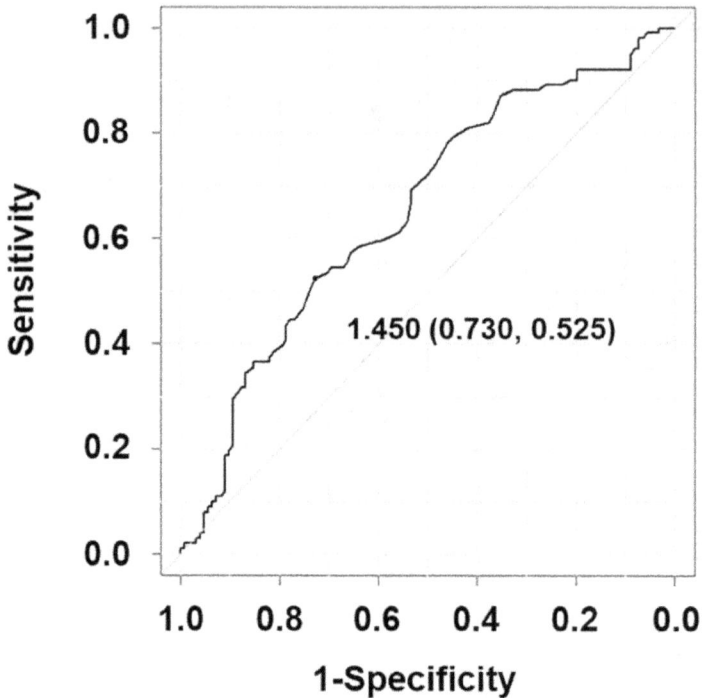

Fig. 1. ROC curve of PT-INR for DIC-related 28-day mortality after rTM treatment.

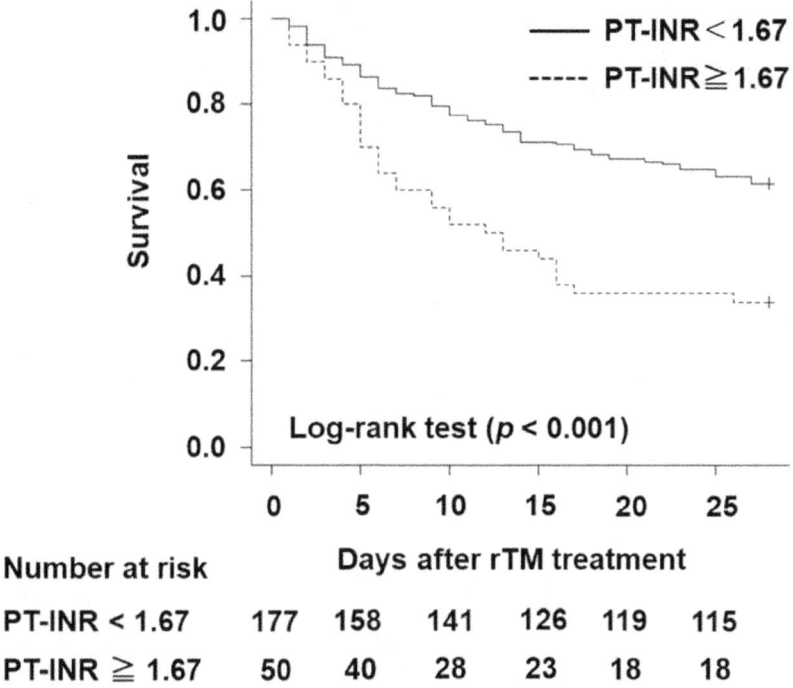

Number at risk

PT-INR < 1.67	177	158	141	126	119	115
PT-INR ≥ 1.67	50	40	28	23	18	18

Fig. 2. 28-day survival curves after rTM in patients with PT-INR ≥ 1.67 and PT-INR < 1.67.

The survival rate of patients with PT-INR ≥ 1.67 was significantly higher than that of patients with PT-INR < 1.67 ($p < 0.001$). PT-INR, prothrombin time-international normalized ratio; rTM, recombinant human soluble thrombomodulin.

Table 1 Diagnostic criteria for DIC by the JAAM scoring system [9]

			Point
SIRS score [10]	Body temperature (°C)	38≦ or <36	
	Respiratory rate	20/min≦	
	Heart rate	90/min≦	
	WBC (/μL)	12,000≦ or ≦4000	
		positive factor 3≦	1
PLT (×10⁴/μL)		8≦ <12	1
		<8	3
PT-INR		1.2≦	1
FDP (μg/mL)		10≦ <25	1
		25≦	3
		DIC is diagnosed when exceeded total of 4 points	

FDP: fibrinogen degradation products. PLT: platelet. PT-INR: prothrombin time-international normalized ratio. SIRS: systemic inflammatory response syndrome. WBC: white blood cell

Table 2 Baseline clinical characteristics and laboratory data of patients

Factors	Survive n = 124	Death n = 103	p value
Sex (Male/Female)	69/55	72/31	0.029[a]
Age	77 (68.5-85.5)[e]	79 (72-87)[e]	0.702[b]
Body weight (kg)	51.3 (45.8-60.0)[e]	48 (42-59)[e]	0.322[b]
eGFR (mL/min/1.73 m^2)	38.5 (16.4-57.3)[e]	42.5 (22.9-69.1)[e]	0.272[c]
Proportion of patients with sepsis-induced DIC (%)	96	93	0.283[a]
Proportion of patients with solid tumor-induced DIC (%)	1.5	4	0.411[a]
Proportion of patients with trauma-induced DIC (%)	2.5	3	1.000[a]
SIRS score	2 (1.0-3.0)[e]	2 (1.0-3.0)[e]	0.226[b]
FDP (µg/mL)	32.5 (19.2-64.8)[e]	41.6 (20.7-77.1)[e]	0.137[c]
PLT (×10^4/µL)	5.6 (3.8-7.7)[e]	5.5 (3.2-7.4)[e]	0.688[c]
PT-INR	1.26 (1.17-1.44)[e]	1.44 (1.28-1.72)[e]	< 0.001[c]
Proportion of patients with warfarin treatment (%)	2.5	1.9	1.000[a]
DIC score[d]	7 (5.8-9.0)[e]	7 (6.0-9.0)[e]	0.365[b]
rTM dose (U/kg)	351 (246-381)[e]	312 (223-381)[e]	0.508[b]
Number of patients treated with ATIII	31	25	1.000[b]
Number of patients treated in ICU	63	39	0.061[a]

eGFR: estimate glomerular filtration rate. SIRS: systemic inflammatory response syndrome. FDP: fibrinogen degradation products. PLT: platelet. PT-INR: prothrombin time-international normalized ratio. ATIII: antithrombin III. ICU: intensive care unit.

[a]Fisher's exact test. [b]Student's t-test. [c]Mann–Whitney U test. [d]JAAM score. [e]Each value represents the median (25%-75% percentile)

Table 3 Cox proportional hazard analysis of some factors of 28-day mortality following rTM treatment.

Factors	Adjusted OR	95% CI	p value
Male	1.66	1.065 – 2.573	0.025
Age ≧ 75	1.57	1.009 – 2.439	0.046
Sepsis-induced DIC	0.32	0.075 – 1.369	0.125
Solid tumor-induced DIC	0.54	0.096 – 3.057	0.487
Trauma-induced DIC	0.45	0.074 – 2.787	0.393
PT-INR ≧ 1.67	2.23	1.451 – 3.433	< 0.001
rTM Dose ≧ 380 U/kg	0.95	0.608 – 1.484	0.820
ATIII co-treatment	0.95	0.598 – 1.501	0.818
Treatment in ICU	0.91	0.595 – 1.380	0.645

OR: odds ratio. 95%CI: 95% confidence interval.

ATIII: antithrombin III. ICU: intensive care unit. PT-INR: prothrombin time-international normalized ratio

Discussion

The 28-day mortality rate after rTM treatment was consistent with those reported in previous studies [8,11]. Although the DIC scores in the survival and death groups were similar, the efficacy of rTM treatment were different. Therefore, we performed Cox regression analysis to elucidate the influential factors.

Elderly patients have reportedly higher mortality rates due to DIC [12]. In this study, we confirmed that the mortality rate was higher for patients over 75 years old than those under 75 years old, indicating that elderly patients have a high mortality rate from DIC even after rTM administration.

According to a previous study, effective blood concentration is not reached unless the dose of rTM is 380 U/kg [13]. Our study showed that the rTM dosage might not be related to efficacy for DIC-related mortality. Further studies are needed to understand the association between blood rTM concentrations and DIC resolution.

Although ROC analysis indicated that the cutoff value of PT-INR was 1.45 (Fig. 1), its clinical relevance is unknown. In the Japanese Ministry of Health and Welfare scoring system, the severity according to PT-INR < 1.25, $1.25 \leq$ PT-

INR < 1.67, and 1.67 ≤ PT-INR are scored as 0, 1, and 2 points, respectively, [2]. Therefore, we selected PT-INR ≥ 1.67 as the cutoff value. Cox regression analysis demonstrated that the 28-day mortality rate in patients with PT-INR ≥ 1.67 was significantly lower than that in patients with PT-INR < 1.67 (Table 3 and Fig. 2), suggesting that PT-INR ≥ 1.67 might be a key factor influencing rTM treatment. The major adverse events occurring in patients with DIC who receive rTM are bleeding-related events [15]. Sugawara *et al.* [15] have suggested that rTM increases the incidence of bleeding-related adverse events, implying that rTM therapy in patients with PT-INR ≥ 1.67 increases the risk of these events. Conversely, an animal study [16] has shown that rTM does not affect the clotting time. Considering our study results, hemorrhage might not affect the 28-day mortality after rTM treatment. A study has revealed that prolonged PT-INR and FDP correlates with DIC severity [2]. Since both severe and mild cases of DIC status were randomly selected in the SCARLET study, the effectiveness of rTM was not proved conclusively [8], suggesting that the rTM treatment for mild DIC status (PT-INR ≥ 1.67) might be effective. However, the value of FDP was not different between the survival and death groups (Table 1), indicating that severe DIC status and other factors related to PT-INR affected rTM efficacy. Warfarin treatment is known to elevate PT-INR [17]. In the present study, because five subjects (three and two subjects from the survival and death groups, respectively) were treated with warfarin (Table 2), their prolonged PT-INR might be influenced by warfarin treatment. Further studies are needed to understand whether prolonged PT-INR directly or indirectly affects DIC-related mortality.

Although male sex was extracted as a factor influencing DIC-mortality after rTM treatment (Table 3), the phenomenon of sex differences has not been reported. Estrogen, a potent steroid hormone present in high levels in females, may have great benefits in anti-inflammation and vascular protection [18]. It is speculated that differences in sex hormones can affect the reactivity of rTM, but further investigation is needed.

Our study design has several limitations. First is the lack of statistical power given the small sample size. Second, because this was a retrospective study, DIC resolution rate could not be evaluated owing to the lack of corresponding information in electronic medical records. Third, non-life-threatening bleeding events, such as gastrointestinal bleeding or intracerebral bleeding, could not be confirmed. Fourth, the underlying diseases in patients were often unknown

19

due to the lack of corresponding information in electronic medical records. Fifth, since the sequential organ failure assessment score was measured only in ICU patients at the Mie Chuo Medical Center from 2019, organ damage was not estimated in the present study.

Conclusions

This study reveals that PT-INR ≥ 1.67, age ≥ 75 years, and male sex may be a factor associated with DIC-related 28-day mortality after rTM treatment. Although the mechanisms underlying the increased mortality rate in patients with PT-INR ≥ 1.67 remain unknown, we proposed that rTM treatment may be less effective in such patients.

References

1. Levi M, and Ten-Cate H. Disseminated Intravascular Coagulation. *N Engl J Med*. 1999; 341:582-592.

2. Wada H, Gabazza-Esteban C, Asakura H, Koike K, Okamoto K, Maruyama I, Shiku H, Nobori T. Comparison of Diagnostic Criteria for Disseminated Intravascular Coagulation (DIC): Diagnostic Criteria of the International Society of Thrombosis and Hemostasis and of the Japanese Ministry of Health and Welfare for Overt DIC. *Am J Hematol*. 2003: 74; 17-22.

3. Weiler H. Regulation of Inflammation by the Protein C System. *Crit Care Med*. 2010: 38; S18-25.

4. Naomi L, Esmon-Whyte G, Esmon-Charles T. Isolation of a Membrane-Bound Cofactor for Thrombin-Catalyzed Activation of Protein C. *J Biol Chem*. 1982: 257; 859-864.

5. Saito H, Maruyama I, Shimazaki S, Yamamoto Y, Aikawa N, Ohno R, Hirayama A, Matsuda T, Asakura H, Nakashima M, Aoki N. Efficacy and Safety of Recombinant Human Soluble Thrombomodulin (ART-123) in Disseminated Intravascular Coagulation: Results of a Phase III,

Randomized, Double-Blind Clinical Trial. *J Thromb Haemost*. 2007: 5; 31-41.

6. Itoh S, Shirabe K, Kohnoe S, Sadanaga N, Kajiyama K, Yamagata M, Anai H, Harimoto N, Ikegami T, Yoshizumi T, Maehara Y. Impact of Recombinant Human Soluble Thrombomodulin for Disseminated Intravascular Coagulation. *Anticancer Res*. 2016: 36; 2493-2496.

7. Yoshihiro S, Sakuraya M, Hayakawa M, Ono K, Hirata A, Takaba A, Kawamura N, Tsutsui T, Yoshida K, Hashimoto Y. Recombinant Human-Soluble Thrombomodulin Contributes to Reduced Mortality in Sepsis Patients With Severe Respiratory Failure: A Retrospective Observational Study Using a Multicenter Dataset. *Shock*. 2019; 51: 174-179.

8. Vincent J L, Francois B, Zabolotskikh I, Kumar-Daga M, Lascarrou J, Kirov-Mikhail Y, Pettilä V, Wittebole X, Meziani F, Mercier E, Lobo-Suzana M, Barie-Philip S, Crowther M, Esmon-Charles T, Fareed J, Gando S, Gorelick-Kenneth J, Levi M, Mira Jean-Paul, Opal-Steveb M, Parrillo J, Russell-James A, Saito H, Tsuruta K, Sakai T, Fineberg D, SCARLET Trial Group. Effect of a Recombinant Human Soluble Thrombomodulin on Mortality in Patients With Sepsis-Associated Coagulopathy: The SCARLET

Randomized Clinical Trial. *JAMA*. 2019; 321: 1993-2002.

9. Gando S, IbavT, Eguchi Y, Ohtomo Y, Okamoto K, Koseki K, Mayumi T, Murata A, Ikeda T, Ishikura H, Ueyama M, Ogura H, Kushimoto S, Saitoh D, Endo S, Shimazaki S, Japanese Association for Acute Medicine Disseminated Intravascular Coagulation (JAAM DIC) Study Group. A multicenter, prospective validation of disseminated intravascular coagulation diagnostic criteria for critically ill patients: comparing current criteria. *Crit Care Med*, 2006; 34: 625-631.

10. Kaukonen K, Bailey M, Pilcher D, Jamie-Cooper D, Bellomo R. Systemic Inflammatory Response Syndrome Criteria in Defining Severe Sepsis. *N Engl J Med.* 2015; 372: 1629-1638.

11. Sawano H, Shigemitsu K, Yoshinaga Y, Tsuruoka A, Natsukawa T, Hayashi Y, Kai T. Combined therapy with antithrombin and recombinant human soluble thrombomodulin in patients with severe sepsis and disseminated intravascular coagulation. *JJAAM*. 2013; 24: 119-131.

12. Banno S, Nitta M, Kikuchi M, Takada K, Mitomo Y, Niimi N, Yamamoto T. Disseminated intravascular coagulation (DIC) and pre-DIC due to severe infection in the elderly. *Nihon Ronen Igakkai Zasshi*, 1994; 31: 747-751.

13. Hayakawa M, Kushimoto S, Watanabe E, Goto K, Suzuki Y, Kotani T, Kiguchi T, Yatabe T, Tagawa J, Komatsu F, Gando S. Pharmacokinetics of recombinant human soluble thrombomodulin in disseminated intravascular coagulation patients with acute renal dysfunction. *Thromb Haemost.* 2017; 117: 851-859.

14. Kanda Y. Investigation of the Freely Available Easy-To-Use Software 'EZR' for Medical Statistics. *Bone Marrow Transplant.* 2013; 48: 452-458.

15. Sugawara J, Suenaga K, Hoshiai T, Sato T, Nishigori H, Nagase S, Yaegashi N. Efficacy of Recombinant Human Soluble Thrombomodulin in Severe Postpartum Hemorrhage With Disseminated Intravascular Coagulation. *Clin Appl Thromb Hemost.* 2013; 19: 557-561.

16. Mohri M, Gonda Y, Oka M, Aoki Y, Gomi K, Kiyota T, Sugihara T, Yamamoto S, Ishida T, Maruyama I. The Antithrombotic Effects of Recombinant Human Soluble Thrombomodulin (rhsTM) on Tissue Factor-Induced Disseminated Intravascular Coagulation in Crab-Eating Monkeys (Macaca Fascicularis). *Blood Coagul Fibrinolysis.* 1997; 8: 274-283.

17. Lutomski D M, Djuric P E, Draeger R W. Warfarin therapy. The effect of heparin on prothrombin times. *Arch Intern Med,* 1987; 147: 432-433.

18. Knowlton A. A. and Lee A. R. Estrogen and the Cardiovascular System.

Pharmacol Ther, 2012; 135: 54-70.

Chapter 2

Combination therapy of midodrine and droxidopa for refractory hypotension in heart failure with preserved ejection fraction per a pharmacist's proposal: a case report

Authors

Yuki Asai, Tomoaki Sato, Daisuke Kito, Takanori Yamamoto, Iwao Hioki, Yasuhisa Urata, Yasuharu Abe

Abstract

Background: Patients with chronic heart failure (CHF) are often treated using many diuretics for symptom relief; however, diuretic use may have to continue despite hypotension development in these patients. Here, we present a case of heart failure with preserved ejection fraction (HFpEF), which is defined as ejection fraction ≥50% in CHF, and refractory hypotension, which was treated with midodrine and droxidopa to normalize blood pressure.

Case presentation: The patient was a 62-year-old man with a history of HFpEF due to mitral regurgitation and complaints of dyspnea on exertion. He had been prescribed multiple medications at an outpatient clinic for CHF management, including azosemide 60 mg/day, bisoprolol 2.5 mg/day, enalapril 2.5 mg/day, spironolactone 50 mg/day, and tolvaptan 15 mg/day. The systolic blood pressure (SBP) of the patient remained at 70–80 mmHg because the use of the diuretic could not be reduced or discontinued owing to edema and weight gain. He was hospitalized for the exacerbation of CHF. Although midodrine 8 mg/day was administered to improve hypotension, the SBP of the patient increased only up to 90 mmHg. On the 35th day after hospitalization, the urine volume decreased significantly (<100 mL/day) due to hypotension. When droxidopa 200 mg/day replaced intravenous noradrenaline on the 47th day, the SBP remained at 100–120 mmHg and the urine volume increased.

Conclusions: Oral combination treatment with midodrine and droxidopa might contribute to the maintenance of blood pressure and diuretic activity in HFpEF patients with refractory hypotension. However, further long-term studies evaluating the safety and efficacy of this combination therapy for patients with HFpEF are needed.

Background

While it is well-known that diuretic treatment is crucial to improve the prognosis and symptoms among patients with chronic heart failure (CHF) [1-3], a diminished diuretic response is common in these patients, increasing the required diuretic dose [4]. Hypotension has been defined as systolic blood pressure (SBP) <90 mmHg and/or diastolic blood pressure (DBP) <60 mmHg [5]. In particular, diuretic-induced hypotension causes dizziness [6]. However, the administration of diuretics in these patients cannot be stopped as this would likely result in the progression of heart failure [7].

Many reports have shown that droxidopa, a noradrenaline (NA) prodrug, improves the symptoms of orthostatic hypotension in patients with Parkinson disease, multiple system atrophy, and pure autonomic failure [8-10]. While extensive evidence is available regarding neurogenic hypotension, information on the efficacy and safety of droxidopa for refractory hypotension with CHF is insufficient. Midodrine is widely used for the management of orthostatic blood pressure [11]; however, there is no evidence available on the efficacy of the combination of midodrine and droxidopa. In recent years, drug treatment has been reported to improve prognosis in heart failure with reduced ejection fraction (HFrEF), in which ejection fraction (EF) is <40% [1-3]. However, guidelines for the treatment of heart failure with preserved ejection fraction (HFpEF), in which EF is ≥50%, are not available. Here, we describe the case of a patient with HFpEF who was successfully treated for refractory hypotension.

Case presentation

The patient was a 62-year-old man with a history of CHF due to mitral regurgitation and complaints of dyspnea on exertion (New York Heart Association functional class III). After mitral annuloplasty, he was prescribed multiple medications at an outpatient clinic for the management of CHF, including azosemide 60 mg/day, bisoprolol 2.5 mg/day, enalapril 2.5 mg/day, spironolactone 50 mg/day, and tolvaptan 15 mg/day. The SBP of the patient remained at 70–80 mmHg because diuretic use could not be reduced or discontinued due to the possible effects of edema and weight gain. He was hospitalized for exacerbation of heart failure. On admission, his SBP and DBP were 83 and 47, respectively, and his heart rate (HR) was 88 beats/min. On the 3rd day after hospitalization, a pharmacist proposed midodrine 4 mg/day, an oral pressor with a weak effect on HR [12], to the attending doctor, after which drug administration was started (Fig. 3). The EF was measured on the 8th day and was 53.4%, which is categorized as HFpEF. Furosemide 20 mg/day was started because the urine volume was low on the 8th day. Over a 9-day period after the initiation of midodrine treatment, the dose was increased to 8 mg/day; however, SBP increased only up to 90 mmHg. Although amezinium 20 mg/day was administered on the 25th day for further pressor action, it was discontinued on the 29th day due to the onset of tachycardia (Fig. 3).

In HFrEF, enalapril has been shown to contribute to improved prognosis [13], whereas it is unknown if this effect is present in HFpEF. However, because in HFpEF it may also be highly beneficial to continue with renin-angiotensin system inhibitors, we changed the drug regimen to losartan, which is reported to have a weak hypertensive effect among the angiotensin II receptor blockers [14]. From the 35th day of hospitalization, blood pressure decreased and urine volume decreased significantly (<100 mL/day), and losartan was discontinued on the 36th day. Consequently, the patient underwent continuous hemodiafiltration (CHDF) on the 36th day only. As shown in Fig. 3, continuous intravenous infusion of dopamine from the 35th day and NA and human atrial natriuretic peptide from the 36th day gradually increased the blood pressure and urine volume. However, it was suggested that it would not be possible to maintain blood pressure upon NA discontinuation. Therefore, the attending doctor consulted a pharmacist regarding the switch from NA to oral pressor drugs. On the basis of some case reports [8-10], the pharmacist suggested switching from intravenous NA to droxidopa, which is converted to NA in vivo, on the 47th day. When the dosage of droxidopa was increased from 200 mg/day to 300 mg/day on the 49th day of hospitalization, SBP and DBP increased to 100–120 mmHg and 60–80 mmHg, respectively. As blood pressure increased, urine volume could be maintained at an average of 3,000 mL/day. Seven days after the start of this combination therapy, the EF was 60.1% (Day 53), and no decrease was observed compared to the findings on the Day 8 (EF = 53.4%). In addition, this combination therapy also did not affect cardiothoracic ratio (CTR) (Day 8: CTR = 58% and Day 60: CTR = 58%) (Fig. 4). After discharge, the patient's SBP and DBP were maintained using a combination of midodrine 8 mg/day and droxidopa 300 mg/day therapy, and his dizziness disappeared.

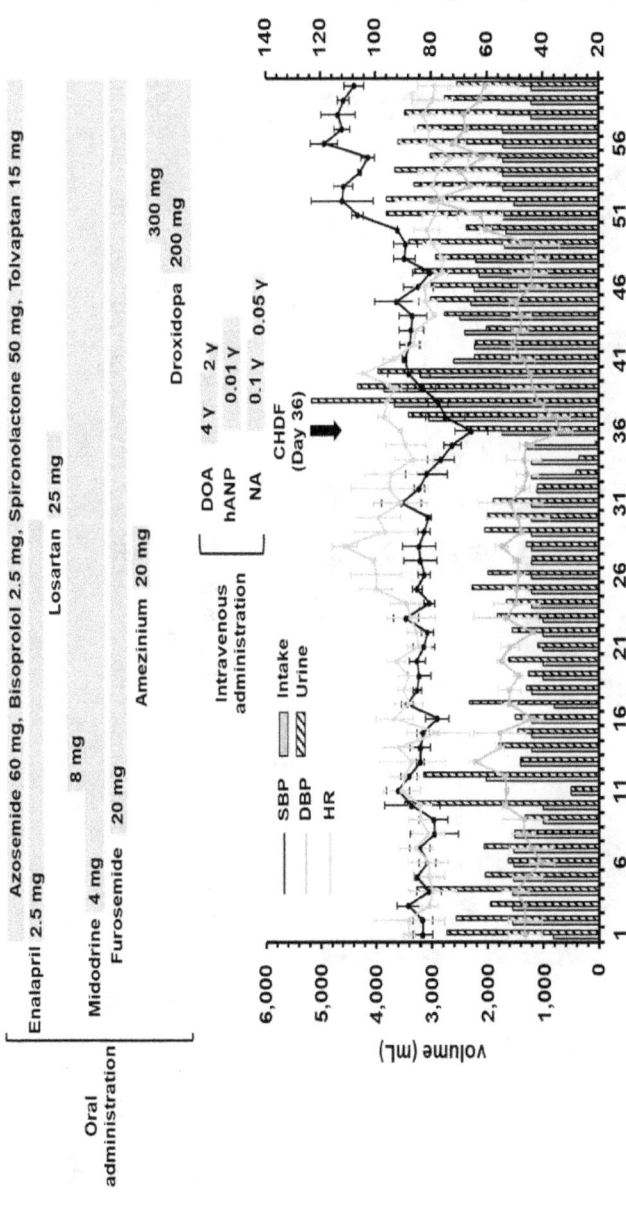

Fig. 3 Clinical course of the hospitalized patient in this study.

Up-titration and down-titration of medications while in the hospital are shown, along with the daily urine volume, intake volume, blood pressure, and HR. BP, blood pressure; CHDF, continuous hemodiafiltration; DBP, diastolic blood pressure; DOA, dopamine; hANP, human atrial natriuretic peptide; HR, heart rate; NA, noradrenaline; SBP, systolic blood pressure. The unit γ shows μg/kg/min. SBP, DBP, and HR are shown as the mean ± standard deviation (SD).

33

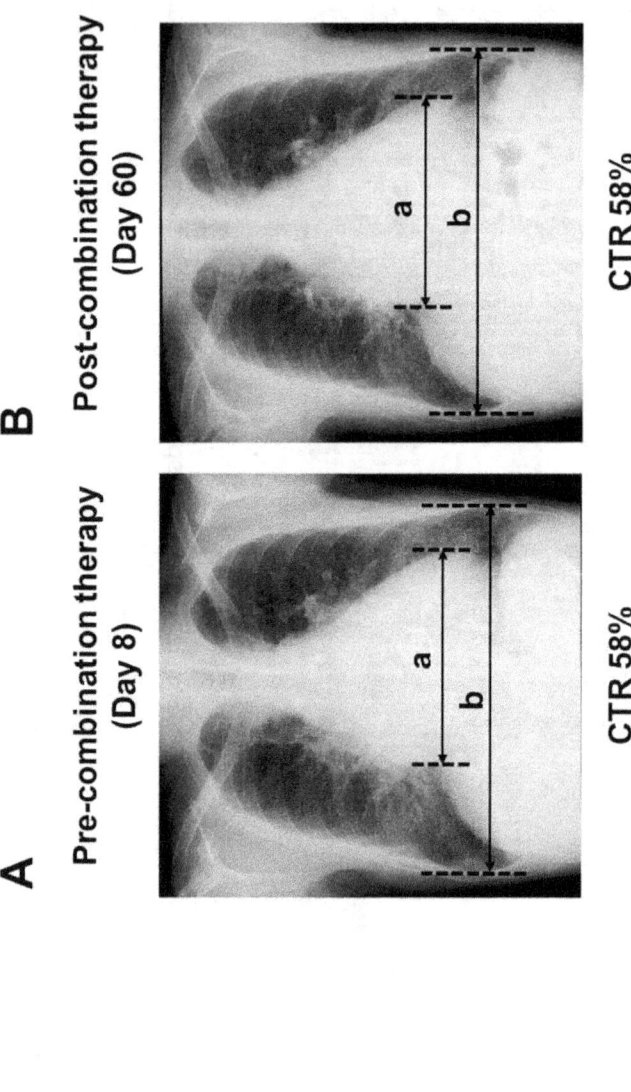

Fig. 4 Chest X-ray of the patient pre- and post-combination therapy with midodrine and droxidopa.

Cardiothoracic ratio (CTR, %) was calculated as (a/b) × 100. (A) Chest X-ray showing pre-combination therapy status on the 8th day of hospitalization with a CTR of 58%. (B) Chest X-ray showing post-combination therapy status on the 60th day of hospitalization with a CTR of 58%.

Discussion and Conclusions

Hypotension is one of the most serious side effects of diuretics in patients with CHF [6]. It causes not only dizziness, but also reduction of diuretic activity because of decreased blood flow [4]. Therefore, it is suggested that improving hypotension may contribute to ensuring diuretic responsiveness. In the case of our patient with HFpEF and refractory hypotension, combination therapy of midodrine and droxidopa increased blood pressure and improved diuretic responsiveness.

While a β-blocker may have potential to improve prognosis in HFpEF [15], bisoprolol decreases blood pressure [16]. In this case, because bisoprolol was used to control tachycardia, we continued to administer bisoprolol at the lowest possible dose while monitoring the HR.

Midodrine is an oral alpha-1 adrenergic agonist that acts as a blood pressor [11] and decreases HR [12]. Although the sample size was small, it was also reported that midodrine elevates EF significantly in HFrEF [17]. Considering this evidence, midodrine might be considered suitable as an oral pressor for patients with HFpEF. Midodrine can elevate SBP and DBP by approximately 20 mmHg [17], and the degree of increase in blood pressure in our patient was similar to that reported previously [17]. Although amezinium was administered on the 25th day, the HR of the patient increased (Fig. 3). Katoh et al. [18] revealed that amezinium elevated HR. Tachycardia is known to be an exacerbating prognostic factor for heart failure [19], suggesting that midodrine, but not amezinium, may show efficacy as an oral pressor in patients with HFpEF.

Despite the administration of midodrine, the urine volume decreased due to excessive hypotension on the 34th and 35th days of hospitalization, and CHDF was performed on the 36th day. It was speculated that the blood pressure might be insufficiently maintained. Because droxidopa is metabolized by L-aromatic-amino-acid decarboxylase to NA, which mediates a pressor response [20], it may be useful to switch from intravenous to oral NA treatment due to hypotension. As expected, up-titration of droxidopa from 200 to 300 mg/day combined with 8 mg/day midodrine rapidly and significantly improved hypotension. Because the blood pressure of the patient could be maintained using this combination therapy, it is considered that the responsiveness to diuretics increased. Therefore, it may be possible to reduce the dose of diuretics such as furosemide. In a double-blind, 4-period crossover study, there were no clinically relevant effects of droxidopa on HR [21]. While the cardiovascular safety of droxidopa has been reported in patients with neurogenic hypotension [22], the detailed safety profile in patients with a history of HFpEF remains unknown. No adverse effects of the combination therapy were noted over the short term in this case. To the best of our knowledge, there is no information regarding the efficacy and safety of droxidopa combined with midodrine in HFpEF patients over the long term. Accordingly, further studies evaluating the safety and efficacy of long-term combination therapy of droxidopa and midodrine for HFpEF patients are needed.

Based on our findings, the combination therapy of midodrine and droxidopa might be safely and effectively administered to HFpEF patients with refractory hypotension, but further studies need to be conducted. In general, diuretic use should be reduced or discontinued if hypotension develops in patients with CHF. If the administration of diuretics must be continued owing to CHF progression, it is advisable to first start midodrine and then add droxidopa if hypotension cannot be effectively controlled.

References

1. Felker GM, Lee KL, Bull DA, David A Bull, Redfield MM, Stevenson LW, Goldsmith SR, LeWinter MM, Deswal A, Rouleau JL, Ofili EO, Anstrom KJ, Hernandez AF, McNulty SE, Velazquez EJ, Kfoury AG, Chen HH, Givertz MM, Semigran MJ, Bart BA, Mascette AM, Braunwald E, O'Connor CM, NHLBI Heart Failure Clinical Research Network. Diuretic strategies in patients with acute decompensated heart failure. Diuretic strategies in patients with acute decompensated heart failure. N Engl J Med. 2011; 364: 797-805.

2. Pitt B, Zannad F, Remme WJ, Cody R, Castaigne A, Perez A, Palensky J, Wittes J. The effect of spironolactone on morbidity and mortality in patients with severe heart failure. Randomized Aldactone Evaluation Study Investigators. N Engl J Med. 1999; 341: 709-717.

3. Pitt B, Remme W, Zannad F, Neaton J, Martinez F, Roniker B, Bittman R, Hurley S, Kleiman J, Gatlin M, Eplerenone Post-Acute Myocardial Infarction Heart Failure Efficacy and Survival Study Investigators. Eplerenone, a selective aldosterone blocker, in patients with left ventricular dysfunction after myocardial infarction. N Engl J Med. 2003; 348: 1309-1321.

4. Valente MAE, Voors AA, Damman K, Veldhuisen DJV, Massie BM, O'Connor

CM, Metra M, Ponikowski P, Teerlink JR, Cotter G, Davison B, Cleland JGF, Givertz MM, Bloomfield DM, Fiuzat M, Dittrich HC, Hillege HL. Diuretic response in acute heart failure: clinical characteristics and prognostic significance. Eur Heart J. 2014; 35: 1284-1293.

5. Mayo Foundation for Medical Education and Research. Low blood pressure (hypotension) - symptoms and causes. 2017 https://www.mayoclinic.org/diseases-conditions/low-blood-pressure/symptomscauses/syc-20355465 Accessed 29 November 2020.

6. Martín-Pérez M, Michel A, Ma M, Rodríguez LAG. Development of hypotension in patients newly diagnosed with heart failure in UK general practice: retrospective cohort and nested case-control analyses. BMJ Open. 2019; 9: e028750.

7. Shah N, Madanieh R, Alkan M, Dogar MU, Kosmas CE, Vittorio TJ. A perspective on diuretic resistance in chronic congestive heart failure. Ther Adv Cardiovasc Dis. 2017;11: 271-278.

8. Kaufmann H, Freeman R, Biaggioni I, Low P, Pedder S, Hewitt LA, Mauney J, Feirtag M, Mathias CJ, NOH301 Investigators. Droxidopa for neurogenic orthostatic hypotension: a randomized, placebo-controlled, phase 3 trial.

Neurology. 2014; 83: 328-335.

9. Hauser RA, Hewitt LA, Isaacson S. Droxidopa in patients with neurogenic orthostatic hypotension associated with Parkinson's disease (NOH306A). J Parkinsons Dis. 2014; 4: 57-65.

10. Isaacson S, Vernino S, Ziemann A, Rowse GJ, Kalu U, White WB. Long-term safety of droxidopa in patients with symptomatic neurogenic orthostatic hypotension. J Am Soc Hypertens. 2016; 10: 755-762.

11. Low PA, Gilden JL, Freeman R, Sheng KN, McElligott MA. Efficacy of midodrine vs placebo in neurogenic orthostatic hypotension. A randomized, double-blind multicenter study. Midodrine Study Group. JAMA. 1997; 277: 1046-1051.

12. Ward CR, Gray JC, Gilroy JJ, Kenny RA. Midodrine: a role in the management of neurocardiogenic syncope. Heart. 1998; 79: 45-49.

13. Yusuf S, Pitt B, Davis CE, Hood Jr WB, Cohn JN. Effect of enalapril on mortality and the development of heart failure in asymptomatic patients with reduced left ventricular ejection fractions. N Engl J Med. 1992; 327: 685-691.

14. Satoh M, Haga T, Hosaka M, Miki Hosaka, Obara T, Metoki H, Murakami T, Kikuya M, Inoue R, Asayama K, Mano N, Ohkubo T, Imai Y. The velocity of

antihypertensive effects of seven angiotensin II receptor blockers determined by home blood pressure measurements. J Hypertens, 2016; 34: 1218-1223.

15. Yancy CW, Lopatin M, Stevenson LW, Marco TD, Fonarow GC, ADHERE Scientific Advisory Committee and Investigators. Clinical presentation, management, and in-hospital outcomes of patients admitted with acute decompensated heart failure with preserved systolic function: a report from the Acute Decompensated Heart Failure National Registry (ADHERE) Database. J Am Coll Cardiol, 2006; 47: 76-84.

Publisher: Eliva Press SRL

Email: info@elivapress.com

Eliva Press is an independent publishing house established for the publication and dissemination of academic works all over the world. Company provides high quality and professional service for all of our authors.

Our Services:
Free of charge, open-minded, eco-friendly, innovational.

-Free standard publishing services (manuscript review, step-by-step book preparation, publication, distribution, and marketing).
-No financial risk. The author is not obliged to pay any hidden fees for publication.
-Editors. Dedicated editors will assist step by step through the projects.
-Money paid to the author for every book sold. Up to 50% royalties guaranteed.
-ISBN (International Standard Book Number). We assign a unique ISBN to every Eliva Press book.
-Digital archive storage. Books will be available online for a long time. We don't need to have a stock of our titles. No unsold copies. Eliva Press uses environment friendly print on demand technology that limits the needs of publishing business. We care about environment and share these principles with our customers.
-Cover design. Cover art is designed by a professional designer.
-Worldwide distribution. We continue expanding our distribution channels to make sure that all readers have access to our books.

www.elivapress.com